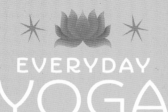

EVERYDAY YOGA

50 POSES FOR HEALING & RELAXATION

JESSIE OLESON MOORE

RP Minis®
Hachette Book Group
1290 Avenue of the Americas, New York, NY 10104
www.runningpress.com
@Running_Press

First Edition: October 2024

Published by RP Minis, an imprint of Hachette Book Group,
Inc. The RP Minis name and logo is a registered trademark of
Hachette Book Group, Inc.

Running Press books may be purchased in bulk for business,
educational, or promotional use. For more information, please
contact your local bookseller or the Hachette Book Group
Special Markets Department at Special.Markets@hbgusa.com.

The publisher is not responsible for websites (or their content)
that are not owned by the publisher.

Design by Amanda Richmond

ISBN: 978-0-7624-8781-3

CONTENTS

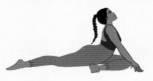

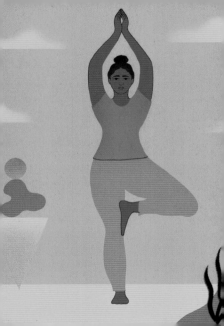

INTRODUCTION

Believe it or not, yoga isn't just an excuse to take a nap or wear overpriced pants (though hey, you look great). The term yoga is derived from the Sanskrit *yuj*, which means "to yoke"—but not in the oxen style. Asana, or the physical practice of yoga, is about harnessing your vital energy by uniting breath and movement. The results can be astounding for your mind and body—so let's wrap this up and get to the postures, shall we?

Note: This guide is intended as an introduction to yoga—these are key postures and productive stretches anyone can add to their daily routine. But there's plenty more nuance to each pose, and there are plenty more poses to discover. I strongly suggest classes at a local studio to put your newfound education to work!

Poses are rated 1-4 stars for general difficulty. All meant for beginners, with 4 stars generally representing the most challenging poses.

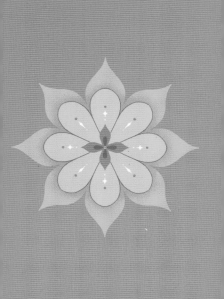

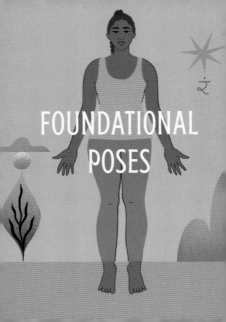

FOUNDATIONAL

POSES

DOWNWARD-FACING DOG ★★

ADHO MUKHA SVANASANA

adhas = "down" · mukha = "face"
svana = "dog" · asana = "posture"

Despite the silly name referring to the pose's resemblance to a dog's waking stretch, downward-facing dog is serious business in the yoga world. To get into this foundational inversion, plant your hands and feet apart on the ground so your body forms a big inverted "V" shape. It strengthens the core, back, and arms, while providing a deep hamstring stretch.

9

CHILD'S POSE ★

BALASANA

bala = "child"

asana = "posture"

This grounding pose, said to be named after its resemblance to a child at rest, is a yoga crowd favorite. Try it: Kneel, with knees together or slightly apart, place your third eye to the ground, and extend your arms forward or backward along your sides. In addition to giving your forehead a mini massage, this pose is a palate cleanser between more active poses.

CORPSE POSE ★

SAVASANA

sava = "corpse"
asana = "posture"

The easiest and *most important* yoga pose—just lie down with your arms at your sides. Despite the macabre name, corpse pose is about integration and renewal: Often the closing posture of a yoga sequence, it lets you absorb the effects of your practice before you rejoin the real world.

TABLE TOP POSE ★

BHARMANASANA
bharma = "table"
asana = "posture"

Get on your hands and knees and marvel as your back becomes a "tabletop" supported by your limbs. Generally, this pose isn't held for very long but acts as a transitional pose/starting point for poses like cat/cow pose or downward-facing dog. Table Top realigns the spine and improves balance.

EASY POSE ★

SUKHASANA

sukham = "ease"
asana = "posture"

To get into this meditative pose, simply assume the posture of a child at story time: Sit up straight, fold your legs, and rest your hands atop your knees (hands down = grounding, hands up = receptive, energizing). The real work here is relaxing: Unclench your jaw, let your spine be loose without slouching, and let your breath flow freely, calming your entire system.

FOUR-LIMBED STAFF POSE ★ ★ ★ ★

CHATURANGA DANDASANA

chatur = "four" • anga = "limb"
danda = "staff" • asana = "posture"

Often referred to as a "yoga push-up," this pose provides full-body toning: Put your full body weight on the hands and feet as your body hovers just above the floor in a plank-like stance, with elbows bent halfway and held close to your body. This pose isn't intended for long holds, it's typically used as a transition between other postures.

MOUNTAIN POSE ★

TADASANA
tada = "mountain"
asana = "posture"

This foundational pose is deceptively simple: It looks like you're just standing up. But it's an *intentional* type of standing. Strongly engage your legs, back, and core, elongate your spine, and let your hands rest open and receptive. Simultaneously strong and expansive, this pose acts as a "home base" in practice as well as a palate cleanser between postures.

PLANK POSE ★ ★ ★

PHALAKASANA

phalaka = "plank"

asana = "posture"

Light as a feather, stiff as a board! To assume this simple but mighty pose, assemble yourself in the upper stance of a push-up, with your full body weight supported by your hands and feet and every part of your body mindfully engaged. (Modify by putting your forearms, knees, or both on the floor.) This posture tones every part of the body and builds balance and endurance.

UPWARD-FACING DOG ★ ★ ★

URDHVA MUKHA SVANASANA
urdhva = "up" • mukha = "face"
svan = "dog" • asana = "posture"

This energizing backbend is
nearly always a transitional pose
in a flow, preceded by downward-
facing dog and four-limbed staff
pose. From the latter, flip forward
onto the tops of your feet, firmly
plant your hands, and arch your
back upward, keeping your thighs
and lower legs lifted. This pose
strengthens the shoulders and
arms and helps combat slouching.

WARRIOR I ★ ★

VIRABHADRASANA

vira = "hero" • bhadra = "friend"
asana = "posture"

Need to swiftly channel your inner warrior? Try this powerful pose (and its companion, Warrior II). Take a wide stance with hips squared, one leg extended forward with bent knee, and the other extended backward with toes at an angle. Exalt your arms skyward. This posture's filled with opposing movements that strengthen the back, core, and legs and stretch the front body.

WARRIOR II ★ ★

VIRABHADRASANA II

vira = "hero" • bhadra = "friend"
asana = "posture"

Finding ease in effort is the
name of the game with this
dynamic pose. It's considered a
companion to Virabhadrasana I,
but with some key differences:
First, your hips are open instead
of squared, and second, your
arms stretch long in either
direction. This mighty pose
strengthens the legs, core, back,
and arms while simultaneously
opening and stretching the hips.

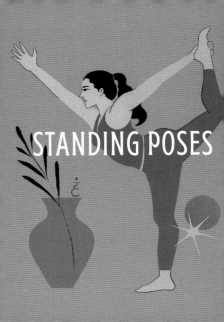

STANDING POSES

CHAIR POSE ★ ★ ★

UTKATASANA

utkata = "powerful"

asana = "posture"

Ever wondered how hard a chair works to hold you up? Try this pose: Assume a "sitting" position with bent knees, but *sans* chair. It's a physical challenge (your legs may wobble!) as well as a mental one ("Get me outta here!"). The payback is building lower body strength and the emotional endurance to better weather life's curveballs.

DANCER POSE ★ ★ ★

NATARAJASANA
nata = "dancer" • raja = "king"
asana = "posture"

Channel your inner ballerina (and challenge your inner balance) with this graceful standing pose. Rest your weight on one leg while extending the other leg behind you with a bent knee. Now, reach your arm back toward the ankle or foot of your raised leg. (Need support? Do it near a wall!) This pose improves balance, strengthens the leg, and stretches your spine.

EXTENDED SIDE ANGLE POSE ★ ★

UTTHITA PARSHVAKONASANA

utthita = "stretch" • parshva = "side"
kona = "angle" • asana = "posture"

Extension is the name of the game
with this fiery posture, which
strengthens your lower body and
stretches your upper limbs, side
body, and spine. To get into it,
assume a Warrior II stance (wide
legs, one knee bent, open hips),
then extend one arm toward the
floor or your extended knee and
reach the other upward at an angle.

GARLAND POSE ★ ★

MALASANA mala = "garland"
asana = "posture"

This wide-knee squat is named for its resemblance to a gently draped necklace, or mala—can you see it? Better yet, try it: Starting from a slightly wider-than-hip-distance stance, bend your knees deeply and bring your bottom almost (but not quite) to the floor. (Use support if needed.) This pose soothes and stretches the lower back and purportedly stimulates the Sacral Chakra, the seat of creativity and sexuality.

LOW LUNGE / CRESCENT LUNGE ★ ★

ANJANEYASANA Anjaneya = "son of Anjani" (Lord Hanuman, the divine entity of spiritual significance) asana = "posture"

This pose takes its name from the mother of a flying monkey (really, look it up). Ready to take the leap? Take a large step forward with one leg, then bend the knee. Keep your back leg up or down and raise your arms toward the sky. This pose stretches the legs and hip flexors, strengthens the thighs and glutes, and can relieve sciatica pain.

PYRAMID POSE ★ ★

PARSVOTTANASANA

parsva = "side" · uttana = "stretch"

asana = "posture"

Make your body a pyramid with this balance-building pose! From a standing position with square hips, one foot steps about three feet forward (semi-wide stance), then you fold forward toward the front knee. Pyramid pose offers a great stretch for your hamstrings and back and improves balance.

STANDING FORWARD BEND ★★

UTTANASANA
uttana = "stretch"
asana = "posture"

Assuming this pose is as straight-forward as its name: From a standing position with feet slightly apart, knees bent or not, reach your upper body down toward the floor. Designed to bring balance between the upper and lower portions of the body, this posture offers an intense hamstring stretch and decompresses the neck and spine.

STANDING SIDE BEND POSE / STANDING HALF MOON POSE ★

PARSVA TADASANA

parsva = "side" • tada = "mountain"
asana = "posture"

If you want to feel a couple of inches taller, try this standing side bend. To get into it, stand up straight (or sit up straight in a chair), reach or clasp the hands overhead, stretch up, then gently extend to one side. (Repeat on the other side.) In addition to stretching the often-ignored side body, this one just feels really good.

TREE POSE ★ ★

VRIKSHASANA

vriksha = "tree" • asana = "posture"

Ever wondered what it's like to
be a tree? Give it a try: Balance
on one leg (your "trunk"). Bend
and lift your other knee and place
your foot above or below the
knee of the standing leg. Stretch
your arms ("branches") overhead
or steeple your palms at heart
center. This posture improves
balance, strengthens stabilizer
muscles in your lower legs, and
builds concentration and focus.

TRIANGLE POSE ★ ★

TRIKONASANA tri = "three"
kona = "corner" or "angle"
asana = "posture"

Translated as "three corners pose," this posture is a trifecta of balance, strength, and flexibility. Configure your limbs into a triangle like so: Open your hips, spread your legs about three feet apart, and extend one arm down toward your front toes. The other arm (and gaze) extends skyward. Triangle pose stretches and lengthens your limbs and spine and helps build balance.

WARRIOR III ★ ★ ★

VIRABHADRASANA

vira = "hero" • bhadra = "friend"
asana = "posture"

Improve your balance,
strengthen your core, and
pretend you're flying all at once!
With Warrior III, you transform
yourself into a fierce T shape like
so: Keep one leg firmly engaged.
The other floats straight back
behind you. Your arms reach
forward. This pose is tough to
hold for long, but it strengthens
the entire body and boosts
concentration.

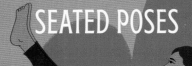

SEATED POSES

BOAT POSE ★ ★ ★

NAVASANA

nava = "boat"

asana = "posture"

Imagine floating serenely at sea—visualization will help because the boat pose can be intense! Fancy a try? Plant your sit bones on the floor, lift your legs till your abs say "Hi!" (fine to balance tiptoes on the ground), and extend your arms forward (gently grasp the legs if desired). As you'll easily feel, this pose is a powerful core, lower back, and quadricep strengthener.

BOW POSE ★ ★ ★

DHANURASANA

dhanu = "bow"
asana = "posture"

Named for its resemblance to a bow (of the arrow variety), this belly-down backbend lifts you up mentally and physically. Using your core and back strength, lift your limbs, expose your beautiful heart to the world, and reach back to grasp your outer ankles. This pose opens your chest, strengthens your spine, and stimulates and helps regulate digestion and your nervous system.

CAT POSE /
COW POSE ★

MARJARIASANA / BITILASANA
marjaria = "cat" • bitila = "cow"
asana = "posture"

Cat and cow poses are paired together so often that flowing between them is considered a single warm-up unit. Start on your hands and knees: for Cow, arch your spine down and look up (mooing is optional). For cat, draw the belly in and up, arch the spine Halloween cat style, and look down. This flow reduces tension in your spine, shoulders, and neck.

COBBLER'S POSE

★ ★ ★

BADDHA KONASANA baddha
= "bound" • kona = "corner" or
"angle" • asana = "posture"

Stretching the inner thighs
and hips can be intense. This
posture, supposedly named for
its resemblance to a cobbler at
work, makes it more accessible.
From seated, bring the soles of
your feet together, bend your
knees, and let them fall outward.
Need support? Blocks or
blankets under the knees work
wonders.

COW FACE POSE

★ ★ ★ ★

GOMUKHASANA

go = "cow" • mukha = "face"

asana = "posture"

Supposedly, your arms resemble a cow's ears and your legs a cow's lips in this awkward seated pose… do you see it? From seated, stack one knee on top of the other with both feet extended toward your sides. Up top, bend one elbow up with the other down and reach your hands together. This challenging pose stretches just about every part of the body.

FROG POSE ★ ★ ★ ★

MANDUKASANA
manduka = "frog"
asana = "posture"

This pose is named for its
resemblance to a peaceful
frog on a lily pad, but it's fairly
intense for most people. Start on
all fours. Lower the forearms to
the ground, then gently spread
the bent knees as far as you
comfortably can in a straddle.
Take it slow, breathe deep, and
enjoy the powerful stretch in your
groin, hips, and inner thighs.

GATE POSE ★★

PARIGHASANA
parigha = "bar" or "beam"

Said to resemble a gate's crossbar, this pose is the "gateway" to stretching your hard-to-reach intercostal (side abdominal) muscles. Do it! Start in an upright kneeling position. Extend one leg long to the side with the foot planted. Use one arm to brace yourself and expand your other arm upward and to the side.

HALF LORD OF THE FISHES POSE ★★

ARDHA MATSYENDRASANA

ardha = "half" • matsya = "fish"
indra = "king" • asana = "posture"

Despite the grand name, inspired by folklore about a fish turned yoga master, this pose is a fairly basic twist. From seated, you bend one knee up and place the foot outside of the other leg, then lift the opposite arm and use it to lever yourself into a deep twist. This pose provides spinal decompression and stimulates digestion.

HAPPY BABY POSE

★ ★

ANANDA BALASANA
ananda = "happiness"
bala = "child" • asana = "posture"

There's no ambiguity behind this posture's name: Just about every baby (happy or not) instinctively assumes this wide-leg posture while lying down. To do it, simply lie on your back, reach for the outside edges of your feet, and gently roll the spine on the floor. This soothing pose gently massages your back, stretches your legs and hips, and just generally feels good.

HEAD-TO-KNEE POSE ★ ★

JANU SIRSASANA
janu = "knee" • sirsa = "head"
asana = "posture"

This pose is just what it sounds like: A seated forward fold where you lean your head down toward (or beyond!) your knee. Take it one leg at a time: Stretch one leg long, bend your other knee, and tuck your foot into the extended leg's inner thigh. Lean forward and try to sniff your knee, stretching the hips and hamstrings.

HERO POSE ★ ★ ★ ★

VIRASANA

vira = "hero"
asana = "posture"

This pose is a real hero for your legs—it stretches them from feet to psoas, including hard-to-stretch muscles around the knees. To get into it, kneel on the floor, raise slightly to peel the calves out from under the thighs, and sit down between your feet (use support if needed). It's an intense stretch. Too much? Go one leg at a time.

PIGEON POSE ★ ★ ★

EKA PADA RAJAKAPOTASANA

eka = "one" • pada = "foot" or
"leg" • raja = "king" • kapota =
"pigeon" • asana = "posture"

This pose, typically held for a
few minutes, offers a mighty
thigh, groin, and psoas stretch,
and is often associated with
emotional release. To get into
it, extend one pigeon wing—er,
leg—forward with your knee
bent out to the side. Bring it to
the floor with your hips squared
and the other leg extending long
behind you. Keep your upper

body upright, or extend forward and down.

Note: Reclining pigeon is a variation where you follow the same movements but from your back.

RECLINING TWIST ★ ★

SUPTA MATSYENDRASANA

supta = "supine" • matsya = "fish"
indra = "king" • asana = "posture"

Named after Matsyendra, a fish
that became an enlightened yogi
(yes, really), this detoxifying twist
relaxes the shoulders and spine,
and also holds the title of "Yoga
pose most likely to accidentally
crack your back." Care to try?
From lying down, draw one knee
in toward your chest, then guide it
across your body. Bring the arms
to a T position, and gaze away
from the bent leg.

SEATED FORWARD BEND ★★

PASCHIMOTTANASANA

paschima = "west" (the direction of the body's back) · uttana = "stretch" asana = "posture"

Guess what? When you were told to "touch your toes" in gym class, you were doing actual yoga. Stretch your legs out long, sit up straight, then extend forward. It's less about bringing your head down to your knees and more about extending your head and spine long toward your toes. You'll feel it most in the hamstrings, but it's a full-body stretch.

SIDE PLANK ★ ★ ★ ★

VASISTHASANA

vasistha = "yogic sage"
asana = "posture"

Quick, somebody snap a pic! To get into this cool-looking pose, start in plank position, then rotate to the side, placing all your body weight on one hand and the blade-edge of the same side. (Modify by putting the weight on the forearm and knee.) Named for the powerful yogi and sage, Vasistha, this pose is rich in benefits. It strengthens the obliques, shoulders, and lats.

WIND-RELIEVING POSE ★★

PAVANA MUKTASANA

pavana = "air/wind"

mukta = "to release"

asana = "posture"

Yep: This posture's name is a shout-out to farting. To get into the pose, you lie down with your legs long. One at a time or both at once, bend your knees and squeeze your legs in tight to your chest. Whether or not you pass gas, the pose can boost digestion and relieve low back pain.

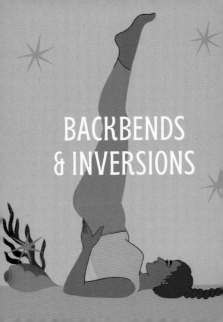

BACKBENDS & INVERSIONS

BRIDGE POSE ★★

SETU BANDHA SARVANGASANA

setu = "bridge" • bandha = "lock"

sarva = "all" • anga = "limb"

asana = "posture"

Is wheel pose just a bit too much?
Take it easier with bridge pose,
a more restorative backbend.
Keeping your head and shoulders
on the ground, lift your knees
and lower back. Bask in the lower
back decompression and leg/glute
strengthening that this pose offers.

CAMEL POSE ★ ★ ★ ★

USTRASANA

ustra = "camel"

asana = "posture"

This potent heart opener may configure you like a camel's hump but acts like an espresso shot for the senses. Start from a kneeling position, then release your head and chest back. Brace your hands on your low back or reach toward your heels (the same motion can be done from the comfort of a chair). This pose increases spinal flexibility and stretches the front body.

COBRA POSE ★ ★

BHUJANGASANA
bhujanga = "cobra"
asana = "posture"

This pose is sometimes used as a modification for upward-facing dog. Start lying down on your belly, draw your hands back to about chest level, and use a combination of your arm and back strength to lift the upper torso off the floor, like a snake lifting its head. This chest-opening pose is a great way to combat "tech neck" and slouching.

DOLPHIN POSE ★ ★ ★

ARDHA PINCHA MAYURASANA
ardha = "half" • pincha = "feather"
mayura = "peacock"
asana = "posture"

This pose is similar to downward-facing dog, but with two important distinctions: 1) Your forearms rest on the ground, and 2) It is named after a sea creature (or a bird, depending on who you ask—in Sanskrit, it's "half-feathered peacock pose"). Either way, it strengthens the entire body including the shoulders.

EXTENDED PUPPY POSE ★★

UTTANA SHISHOSANA

uttana = "stretch" · shishu = "baby"
(dog or puppy) · asana = "posture"

The best parts of downward-
facing dog and child's pose come
together in this mild inversion and
powerful yet gentle heart opener
that stretches your chest, arms, and
spine. Wanna try? Start on all fours,
and extend your front body forward
and down, bringing your chest
toward (or all the way to) the ground.
Your forehead rests on the floor, and
your arms extend forward.

HEADSTAND ★ ★ ★ ★

SALAMBA SHIRSHASANA

salamba = "supported" · shirsha = "head" · asana = "posture"

This pose helps your brain breathe! Flipping upside down delivers a fresh, oxygen-rich flow of blood to your head, improves balance, and gives you a serious core workout. But it takes practice: Support your body weight on your forearms, walk your toes forward, and then lift them into the air. (Just starting? Using a wall behind you for support is strongly encouraged.)

LEGS AGAINST THE WALL ★

VIPARITA KARANI
viparita = "inverted/reversed"
karani = "action"

This is one of yoga's loveliest poses. For this inversion pose, lie down near a wall, raise your legs up, and shimmy your bum as close to the wall as you'd like. From there, all you've got to do is relax. This restorative pose helps lower the heart rate, decrease blood pressure levels, and improve circulation.

LOCUST POSE ★ ★ ★ ★

SALABHASANA

salabha = "locust"
asana = "posture"

This challenging backbend, said
to resemble a grasshopper, is
easy to understand—from a belly-
down position with arms at your
sides and legs long behind you,
you channel your core strength
to lift everything you can. It's not
easy to hold this pose for long, but
try 3–5 breaths, because it's great
for building up spinal flexibility
and strength.

SHOULDER STAND

★ ★ ★

SALAMBA SARVANGASANA
salamba = "supported"
sarvanga = "whole body"
asana = "posture"

All hail the "Queen of all Asanas"—so
nicknamed for its myriad benefits,
including improved circulation,
reduced anxiety, and better digestion.
This inversion is easier than it looks:
From your back, lift your legs, shift
the weight to your shoulders (use a
blanket for support if needed), use
your hands to brace your back, and
bring your legs perpendicular.

THREAD THE NEEDLE POSE ★ ★

SUCIRANDHRASANA

suci = "needle" · randhra = "loop"
asana = "posture"

Your body is both the thread and
the needle in this gentle inversion!
Start on your hands and knees,
and raise one arm up to the side,
opening your chest. Then "thread"
it like a needle between your
other arm and knee. If desired,
extend the front arm forward. This
pose provides a wonderful stretch
for hard-to-reach spots like your
shoulders, upper back, and neck.

WHEEL POSE / UPWARD BOW POSE

★ ★ ★

URDVHA DHANURASANA

urdvha = "up" • dhanu = "bow"
asana = "posture"

Wheel pose, also called upward
bow pose, this is both an inversion
and a backbend that strengthens
the entire body. Start lying down.
Bend your knees and plant your
feet on the floor, then bend the
elbows and place your hands next
to your head. Now, hoist your body
up into a big rainbow shape and
enjoy a big rush of energy!

WIDE-LEG STANDING FOLD ★★

PRASARITA PADOTTANASANA

prasarita = "expanded"
pada = "foot" or "leg"
uttana = "stretch"
asana = "posture"

This simple inversion is easy to master—simply step both feet hip distance apart or wider, and fold forward to your comfort level. The variations are infinite: For one, step the feet closer or wider to stretch different parts of the leg. Clasp the back of your head in your hands for a delightful neck traction stretch for one variation. This posture offers a full body stretch and calms the mind.

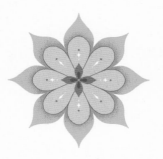

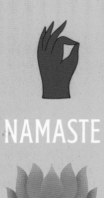

NAMASTE